# Ultimate Air Fryer Cooking Guide

## A Collection of Air Fryer Recipes for All Tastes

By Samantha Hendrick

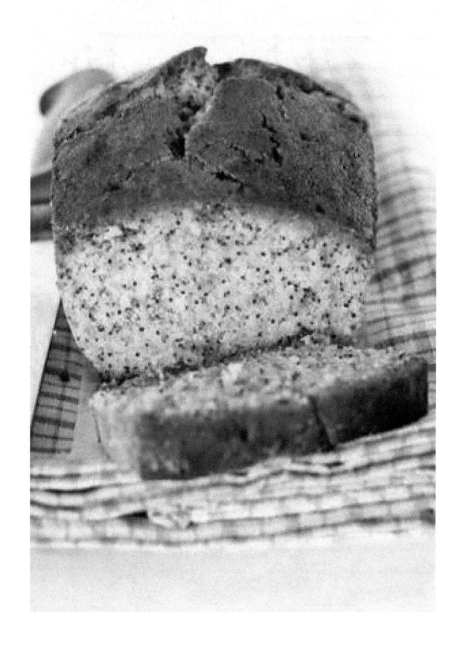

The content within this book has been derived from various sources. Please consult a licensed professional before attempting any techniques outlined in this book.

By reading this document, the reader agrees that under no circumstances is the author responsible for any losses, direct or indirect, which are incurred as a result of the use of information contained within this document, including, but not limited to, — errors, omissions, or inaccuracies.

# Table of Contents

# Peppery Lemon-Chicken Breast

**Serves:** 1

**Cooking Time:**

**Ingredients:**

- 1 chicken breast
- 1 teaspoon minced garlic /5G
- 2 lemons, rinds and juice reserved
- Salt and pepper to taste

**Instructions:**

1) Preheat mid-air fryer.
2) Place all ingredients in a baking dish that will fit within the air fryer.
3) Place inside the air fryer basket.
4) Close and cook for 20 minutes at 400° F or 205°C .

**Nutrition information:**

- Calories per serving: 539
- Carbohydrates: 11.8g
- Protein: 61.8g
- Fat: 27.2g

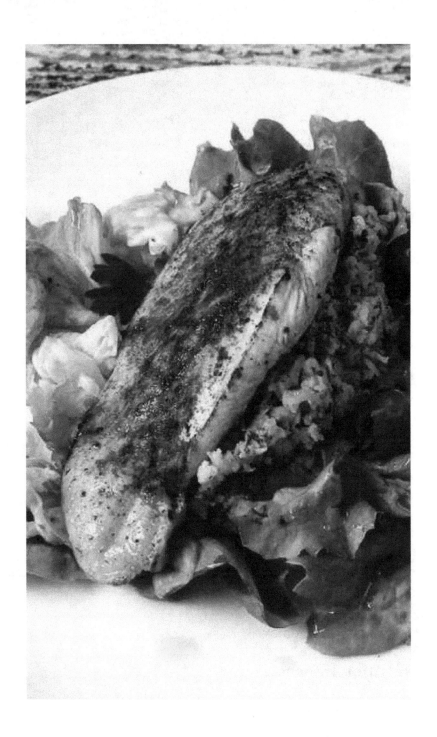

# Pineapple Juice-Soy Sauce Marinated Chicken

**Servings per Recipe:** 5

**Cooking Time:** 20 Minutes

## Ingredients:

- 3 tablespoons light soy sauce /45ML
- 1-pound chicken white meat tenderloins or strips /450G
- 1/2 cup pineapple juice /125ML
- 1/4 cup packed brown sugar /32.5G

## Instructions:

1) Boil pineapple juice, brown sugar, and soy sauce. Transfer to a large bowl. Stir in chicken and pineapple. Let it marinate in the fridge for an hour or more.
2) Thread pineapple and chicken alternatively in skewers. Place on skewer rack.
3) For 10 minutes, cook on 360° F or 183°C . Halfway through cooking time, turnover chicken and baste with marinade.
4) Serve and enjoy.

## Nutrition Information:

- Calories per Serving: 157
- Carbs: 14.7g

- Protein: 19.4g
- Fat: 2.2g

# Quick 'n Easy Brekky Eggs 'n Cream

**Serves:** 2

**Cooking Time:** 15 minutes

## Ingredients:

- 2 eggs
- 2 tablespoons coconut cream /30ML
- A dash of Spanish paprika
- Salt and pepper to taste

## Instructions:

1) Preheat mid-air fryer for 5 minutes.
2) Place the eggs and coconut cream in a bowl. Season with salt and pepper to taste then whisk until fluffy.
3) Pour into greased pan and sprinkle with Spanish paprika.
4) Place in the air fryer.
5) Bake for 15 minutes at 350° F or 177°C .

## Nutrition information:

- Calories per serving:178.1
- Carbohydrates: 1.1g
- Protein: 9.9g
- Fat: 14.9g

# Buttered Spinach-Egg Omelet

**Serves:** 4

**Cooking Time:** 15

**Ingredients:**

- ¼ cup coconut milk /62.5ML
- 1 tablespoon melted butter /15ML
- 1-pound baby spinach, chopped finely /450G
- 3 tablespoons organic olive oil /45G
- 4 eggs, beaten
- Salt and pepper to taste

**Instructions**

1) Preheat the air fryer for 5 minutes.
2) In a mixing bowl, combine the eggs, coconut milk, olive oil, and butter until well-combined.
3) Add the spinach and season with salt and pepper to taste.
4) Pour all ingredients into the baking dish.
5) Bake at 350° F or 177°C for 15 minutes.

**Nutrition information:**

- Calories per serving: 310
- Carbohydrates: 3.6g
- Protein: 13.6g
- Fat: 26.8g

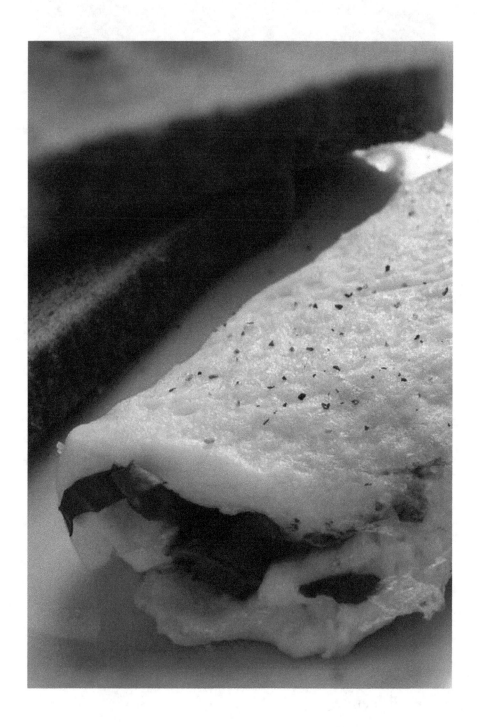

# Caesar Marinated Grilled Chicken

**Servings per Recipe:** 3

**Cooking Time:** 24 minutes

## Ingredients:

- ¼ cup crouton /32.5G
- 1 teaspoon lemon zest. Form into ovals, skewer and grill. /5G
- 1/2 cup Parmesan /65G
- 1/4 cup breadcrumbs /32.5G
- 1-pound ground chicken /450G
- 2 tablespoons Caesar dressing and more for drizzling /30G
- 2-4 romaine leaves

## Instructions:

1) Add chicken, 2 tablespoons Caesar dressing, parmesan, and breadcrumbs to a bowl. Mix well with hands. Use hands to form 1-inch oval patties.
2) Skewer chicken pieces. Place on skewer rack in the air fryer.
3) For 12 minutes, cook on 360° F or 183°C . After 6 minutes, turnover skewers. If needed, cook in batches.
4) Serve, dress with lettuce and sprinkle with croutons and additional dressing. Enjoy.

## Nutrition Information:

- Calories per Serving: 339
- Carbs: 9.5g
- Protein: 32.6g
- Fat: 18.9g

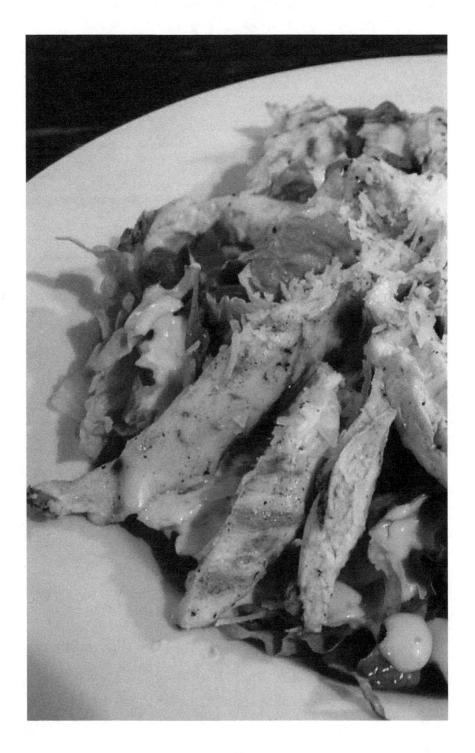

# Cheese Stuffed Chicken

**Servings per Recipe:** 4

**Cooking Time:** 30 Minutes

## Ingredients:

- 1 tablespoon creole seasoning /15G
- 1 tablespoon organic olive oil /15ML
- 1 teaspoon garlic powder /5G
- 1 teaspoon onion powder /5G
- 4 chicken breasts, butterflied and pounded
- 4 slices Colby cheese
- 4 slices pepper jack cheese

## Instructions:

1) Preheat the air fryer to 390° F or 199°C .
2) Place the grill pan accessory in the mid-air fryer.
3) Mix the creole seasoning, garlic powder, and onion powder in a bowl. Season with salt and pepper if desired.
4) Lavishly polish the seasoning on the chicken.
5) Place the chicken on a flat surface and add a slice of pepper jack and Colby cheese.
6) Fold the chicken and secure the sides with toothpicks.
7) Brush chicken with organic olive oil.
8) Grill for 30 minutes and turn over the meat every 10 minutes.

## Nutrition information:

- Calories per serving: 727
- Carbs:5.4 g
- Protein: 73.1g
- Fat: 45.9g

# Cheesy Potato, Broccoli 'n Ham Bake

**Servings per Recipe:** 3

**Cooking Time:** 35 minutes

**Ingredients:**

- 1 1/2 tablespoon mayonnaise /22.5G
- 1/3 cup canned condensed cream of mushroom soup /83ML
- 1/3 cup grated Parmesan cheese /43G
- 1/3 cup milk /83ML
- 3/4 cup 3/cooked, cubed ham /88G
- 6-ounce frozen chopped broccoli /180G
- 6-ounce frozen French fries /180G

**Instructions:**

1) Lightly grease baking pan of air fryer with cooking spray.
2) Evenly spread French fries at the base of the pan. Place broccoli on the top and then evenly spread ham.
3) Add mayonnaise, milk, and soup to a bowl and then pour the mixture over the fries.
4) Sprinkle cheese, cover the pan with a foil.
5) For 25 minutes, cook on 390° F or 199°C . Remove foil and continue cooking for the next 10 minutes.
6) Serve and enjoy.

## Nutrition Information:

- Calories per Serving: 511
- Carbs: 34.7g
- Protein: 22.8g
- Fat: 31.2g

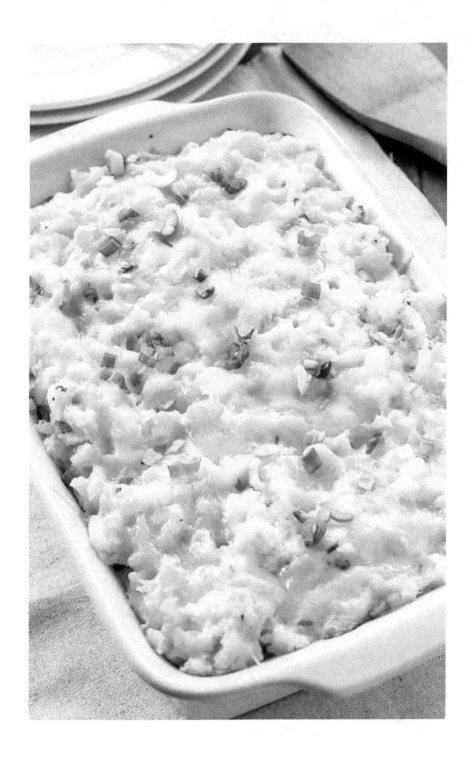

# Cheesy Turkey-Rice with Broccoli

**Servings per Recipe:** 4

**Cooking Time:** 40 minutes

**Ingredients:**

- 1 cup cooked, chopped turkey meat /130G
- 1 tablespoon and 1-1/2 teaspoons butter, melted /22.5ML
- 1/2 (10 ounces) package frozen broccoli, thawed /300G
- 1/2 (7 ounces) package whole-wheat crackers, crushed /210G
- 1/2 cup shredded Cheddar cheese /65G
- 1/2 cup uncooked white rice /65G

**Instructions:**

1) Add two cups of water to a saucepan. Bring to a boil. Add rice, stir and allow to simmer for 20 minutes. Turn off the flame and put it aside.
2) Lightly grease baking pan of air fryer with cooking spray. Add cooked rice and stir. Add cheese, broccoli, and turkey. Mix well to combine.
3) Mix the melted butter and crushed crackers inside a small bowl. Evenly spread this mixture on top of the rice.
4) Cook at 360° F 183°C for 20 minutes or until the tops are lightly browned.
5) Serve and enjoy.

## Nutrition Information:

- Calories per Serving: 269
- Carbs: 23.7g
- Protein: 17.0g
- Fat: 11.8g

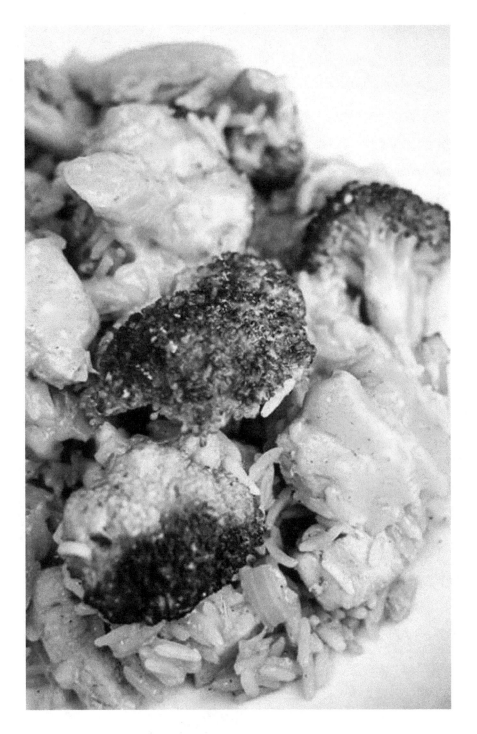

# Gingery Cod Filet Recipe from Hong Kong

**Serves**: 2

**Cooking Time**: 15

**Ingredients:**

- 2 cod fish fillets
- 250 mL water
- 3 tablespoons coconut aminos /45g
- 3 tablespoons coconut oil /45ml
- 5 slices of ginger
- A dash of sesame oil
- Green onions for garnish

**Instructions**:

1) Warm-up air fryer for 5 minutes.
2) Place all ingredients in a baking dish except the green onions.
3) Place in the air fryer and cook for 15 minutes at 4000 F or 205°C .
4) Dress with green onions.

**Nutrition information:**

- Calories per serving: 571
- Carbohydrates: 4.3g

- Protein: 22.3g
- Fat: 51.6g

# Grilled Bacon 'n Scallops

**Servings per Recipe**: 2

**Cooking Time**: 12 minutes

**Ingredients**:

- 1 teaspoon smoked paprika /5g
- 6 bacon strips
- 6 large scallops

**Instructions**:

1) Wrap each bacon around a scallop and thread on a skewer.
2) Season with paprika.
3) Place on skewer rack in the air fryer.
4) Cook for 12 minutes at 3900 F or 199°C . Turnover skewers regularly while cooking.
5) Serve and enjoy.

**Nutrition Information:**

- Calories per Serving: 72
- Carbs: 2.4g
- Protein: 1.9g
- Fat: 6.0g

# Grilled Scallops with Pesto

**Servings per Recipe**: 3

**Cooking Time**: 15

## Ingredients:

- ½ cup prepared commercial pesto /45ml
- 12 large scallops, side muscles removed
- Salt and pepper to taste

## Instructions:

1) Place all ingredients in a Ziploc bag. Place in a fridge to marinate for some hours.
2) Preheat air fryer to 3900 F or 199°C .
3) Place the grill pan in the air fryer.
4) Grill the scallops for 15 minutes.
5) Serve with pasta or bread (optional).

## Nutrition information:

- Calories per serving: 137
- Carbs: 7.7g
- Protein:15.3 g
- Fat: 5g

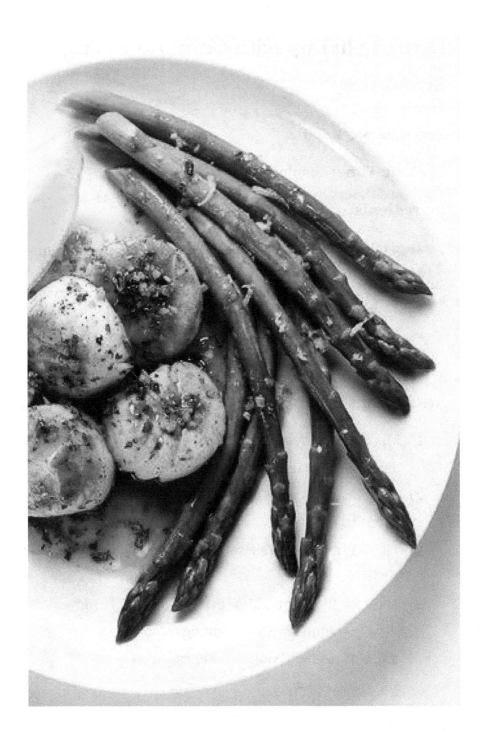

# Grilled Shrimp with Chipotle-Orange Seasoning

**Servings per Recipe**: 2

**Cooking Time**: 24 minutes

**Ingredients:**

- 3 tablespoons minced chipotles in adobo sauce/45ml
- salt
- ½-pound large shrimps /225g
- juice of 1/2 orange
- 1/4 cup barbecue sauce /62.5ml

**Instructions**

1) Mix all ingredients in a shallow bowl except the shrimp. Save one-quarter of the mixture for basting.
2) Add shrimp to a bowl and stir well to coat. Marinate for about 10 minutes.
3) Thread shrimps on skewers. Place on skewer rack in the air fryer.
4) Cook for 12 minutes at 3600 F or 183°C . Turnover skewers regularly while cooking. Also, saturate with sauce. If needed, cook in batches.
5) Serve and enjoy.

**Nutrition Information:**

- Calories per Serving: 179
- Carbs: 24.6g
- Protein: 16.6g
- Fat: 1.5g

# Grilled Squid with Aromatic Sesame Oil

**Servings per Recipe**: 3

**Cooking Time**: 10 minutes

**Ingredients:**

- 1 ½ pounds squid, cleaned /675g
- 2 tablespoons toasted sesame oil /30ml
- Salt and pepper to taste

**Instructions**:

1) Preheat air fryer to 3900 F or 199°C .
2) Place the grill pan in the air fryer.
3) Season the squid with sesame oil, salt and pepper.
4) Grill the squid for 10 minutes.

**Nutrition information:**

- Calories per serving: 220
- Carbs: 0.9g
- Protein: 27g
- Fat: 12g

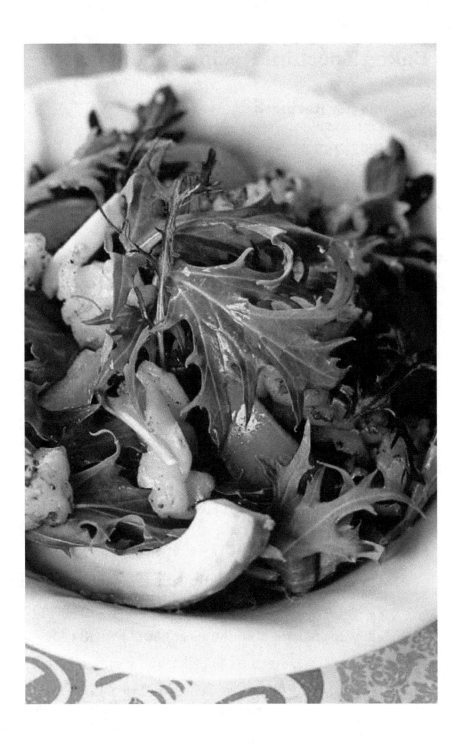

# Baked Zucchini Recipe From Mexico

**Servings per Recipe:** 4

**Cooking Time:** 30 minutes

## Ingredients:

- 1 tablespoon olive oil /15ML
- 1-1/2 pounds zucchini, cubed /675G
- 1/2 cup chopped onion /65G
- 1/2 teaspoon garlic salt /2.5G
- 1/2 teaspoon paprika /2.5G
- 1/2 teaspoon dried oregano /2.5G
- 1/2 teaspoon cayenne pepper, or to taste /2.5G
- 1/2 cup cooked long-grain rice /65G
- 1/2 cup cooked pinto beans /65G
- 1-1/4 cups salsa /195G
- 3/4 cup shredded Cheddar cheese /88G

## Instructions:

1) Spray the baking pan lightly with any oil of your choice to grease it. Drop in onions and zucchini in the pan and allow to cook for 10 minutes at 360O F or 183°C .
2) Add cayenne, oregano, paprika, garlic salt and stir.
3) While stirring add salsa, beans, and rice. Cook for 5 minutes.
4) Also add cheddar cheese and stir well.

5) Cover the pan with aluminium foil.

6) Let it cook for 15 minutes at 390 **O** F or 199°C .

7) Serve and enjoy.

## Nutrition Information:

- Calories per Serving: 263
- Carbs: 24.6g
- Protein: 12.5g
- Fat: 12.7g

# Banana Pepper Stuffed with Tofu 'n Spices

**Serves:** 8

**Cooking Time:** 10 minutes

**Ingredients:**

- ½ teaspoon red chili powder /2.5G
- ½ teaspoon turmeric powder /2.5G
- 1 onion, finely chopped
- 1 package firm tofu, crumbled
- 1 teaspoon coriander powder /5G
- 3 tablespoons coconut oil /15ML
- 8 banana peppers, top quality sliced and seeded
- Salt to taste

**Instructions:**

1) Allow mid-air fryer to warm up for 5 minutes.
2) Add the tofu, onion, coconut oil, turmeric powder, red chili powder, coriander powder, and salt to a mixing bowl. Stir well until properly combined.
3) Using a spoon take a portion of the tofu mixture and place it in the holes of the banana peppers.
4) Place the stuffed peppers in the air fryer.
5) Allow cooking for 10 Minutes at 325° F or 163°C .

## Nutrition information:

- Calories per serving: 72
- Carbohydrates: 4.1g
- Protein: 1.2g
- Fat: 5.6g

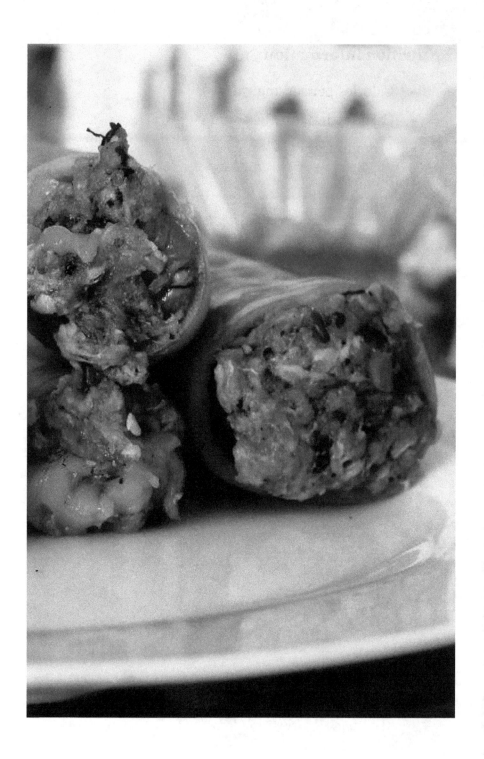

# Bell Pepper-Corn Wrapped in Tortilla

**Serves:** 4

**Cooking Time:** 15

**Ingredients:**

- 1 small red bell pepper, chopped
- 1 small yellow onion, diced
- 1 tablespoon water /15ML
- 2 cobs grilled corn kernels
- 4 large tortillas
- 4 pieces commercial vegan nuggets, chopped
- mixed greens for garnish

**Instructions:**

1) Warm up the air fryer to 400° F or 205°C .
2) Sauté the onions, bell peppers, and corn kernels using water over medium heat in a pan. Set aside.
3) Place filling inside corn tortillas.
4) Fold the tortillas and put them inside a mid-air fryer and cook for 15 minutes before the tortilla wraps are crispy.
5) Serve with mixed greens ahead.

**Nutrition information:**

- Calories per serving: 548
- Carbohydrates: 43.54g

- Protein: 46.73g
- Fat: 20.76g

# Black Bean Burger with Garlic-Chipotle

**Servings per Recipe:** 3

**Cooking Time:** 20 minutes

**Ingredients:**

- ½ cup corn kernels /65G
- ½ teaspoon chipotle powder /2.5G
- ½ teaspoon garlic powder /2.5G
- ¾ cup salsa /88G
- 1 ¼ teaspoon chili powder /6.25G
- 1 ½ cup rolled oats /195G
- 1 can black beans, rinsed and drained
- 1 tablespoon soy sauce /15ML

**Instructions:**

1) Add all ingredients to a mixing bowl and mix using your hands.
2) Make small lumps of the constituent with your hands and hang upside down.
3) Polish the pastry lump with oil (Optional).
4) Place the grill pan in the air fryer and place the pastry lump in the pan.
5) Cook for 20 minutes on both sides at 330° F or 166°C . Ensure both sides are evenly brown.

**Nutrition information:**

- Calories per serving: 395
- Carbs: 52.2g
- Protein: 24.3g
- Fat: 5.8g

# Hollandaise Topped Grilled Asparagus

**Servings per Recipe:** 6

**Cooking Time:** 15 minutes

## Ingredients:

- ¼ teaspoon black pepper /1.25G
- ½ cup butter, melted /125ML
- ½ lemon juice
- ½ teaspoon salt /2.5G
- ½ teaspoon salt /2.5G
- 1 teaspoon chopped tarragon leaves /2.5G
- 2 tablespoons essential olive oil /30ML
- 3 egg yolks
- 3 pounds asparagus spears, trimmed /1350G
- A pinch of mustard powder
- A punch of ground white pepper

## Instructions:

1) Preheat the air fryer to 330° F or 166°C .
2) Place the grill pan in the air fryer.
3) Mix the asparagus, essential olive oil, salt and pepper in a Ziploc bag and shake properly.
4) Place on the grill pan and cook for 15 minutes.

5) Place the double boiler over medium heat, whisk the egg yolks, squeezed fresh lemon juice, and salt until silky. Add the mustard powder, white pepper and melted butter. Keep whisking until the sauce is smooth. Garnish with tarragon leaves.

6) Sprinkle the sauce over asparagus spears.

## Nutrition information:

- Calories per serving: 253
- Carbs: 10.2g
- Protein: 6.7g
- Fat: 22.4g

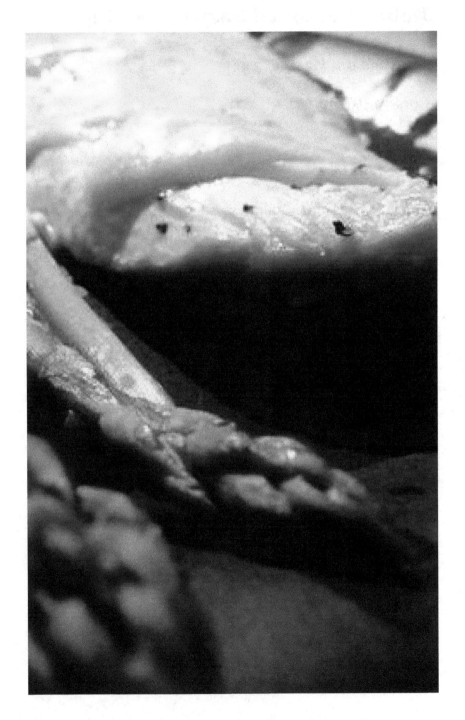

# Italian Seasoned Easy Pasta Chips

**Servings per Recipe:** 2

**Cooking Time:**10

**Ingredients:**

- ½ teaspoon salt /2.5G
- 1 ½ teaspoon Italian seasoning blend /7.5G
- 1 tablespoon nutritional yeast /15G
- 1 tablespoon extra virgin olive oil /15ML
- 2 cups whole wheat bowtie pasta /260G

## Instructions

1) Place the baking dish in a mid-air fryer.
2) Stir all the ingredients together and place them in the baking dish.
3) Close mid-air fryer and cook for 10 minutes at 390° F or 199°C .

## Nutrition information:

- Calories per serving:407
- Carbs: 47g
- Protein: 17.9g
- Fat: 17.4g

# Jackfruit-Cream Cheese Rangoon

**Servings per Recipe:** 2

**Cooking Time:** 10 minutes

**Ingredients:**

- ¾ Thai curry paste /188ML
- 1 can green jackfruit in brine
- 1 cup vegan cream cheese /130G
- 1 scallion, chopped
- 2 cups vegetable broth /500ML
- 2 teaspoon sesame oil /10ML
- Salt and pepper to taste

**Instructions:**

1) Place the baking pan in the air fryer.
2) Add the rest of the ingredients and stir well.
3) Close the air fryer and cook for 10 minutes at 390° F or 199°C .

**Nutrition information:**

- Calories per serving: 457
- Carbs: 107.3g
- Protein: 0.8g
- Fat: 6.8g

# Jalapeno Stuffed with Bacon 'n Cheeses

**Serves:** 8

**Cooking Time:** 15 minutes

**Ingredients:**

- ¼ cup cheddar cheese, shredded /32.5G
- 1 teaspoon paprika /5G
- 16 fresh jalapenos, sliced lengthwise and seeded
- 16 strips of uncured bacon, cut into half
- 4-ounce cream cheese /120G
- Salt to taste

**Instructions:**

1) Mix the cream cheese, cheddar cheese, salt, and paprika in a bowl until well-combined.
2) Put half a teaspoon onto each half of jalapeno peppers.
3) Wrap a thin strip of bacon across the cheese-filled jalapeno half. Put on gloves when doing this because jalapeno is quite spicy.
4) Place in mid-air fryer basket and cook for 15 minutes in a 350° F or 177°C preheated air fryer.

**Nutrition information:**

- Calories per serving: 225
- Carbohydrates: 3.2g

- Protein: 10.6g
- Fat: 18.9g

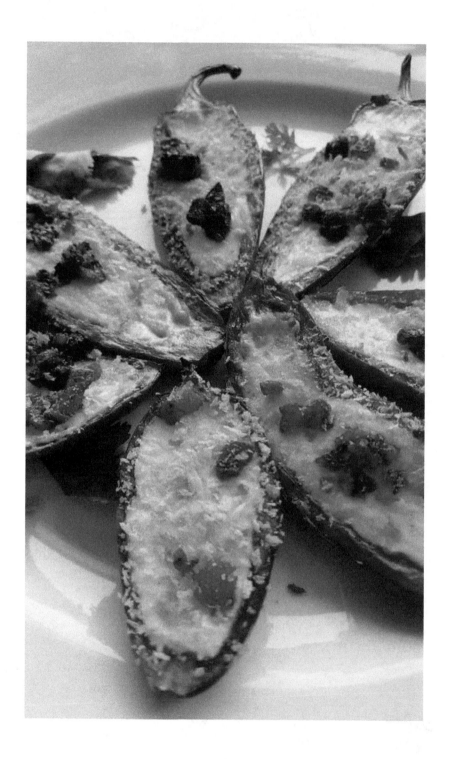

# Layered Tortilla Bake

**Servings per Recipe:** 6

**Cooking Time:** 30 Minutes

**Ingredients:**

- 1 (15 ounces) can black beans, rinsed and drained /450G
- 1 cup salsa /130G
- 1 cup salsa, divided /130G
- 1/2 cup chopped tomatoes /65G
- 1/2 cup sour cream /125ML
- 2 (15 ounces) cans pinto beans, drained and rinsed /450G
- 2 cloves garlic, minced
- 2 cups shredded reduced-fat Cheddar cheese /260G
- 2 tablespoons chopped fresh cilantro /30G
- 7 (8 inches) flour tortillas

**Instructions:**

1) Mash pinto beans in a large bowl and mix in garlic and salsa.
2) Mix tomatoes, black beans, cilantro, and ¼ cup salsa in a bowl.

3) Grease baking pan of air fryer with cooking spray. Spread 1 tortilla, spread ¾ cup pinto bean mixture evenly approximately ½-inch away from the edge of tortilla, spread ¼ cup cheese ahead. Cover with another tortilla spread 2/3 cup black bean mixture after which ¼ cup cheese. Repeat the layering. Cover with the last tortilla, top with pinto bean mixture then cheese.

4) Cover the pan with foil.

5) Cook for 25 minutes at 390° F or 199°C , remove foil and cook for 5 minutes or until tops are lightly browned.

6) Serve and get.

## Nutrition Information:

- Calories per Serving: 409
- Carbs: 54.8g
- Protein: 21.1g
- Fat: 11.7g

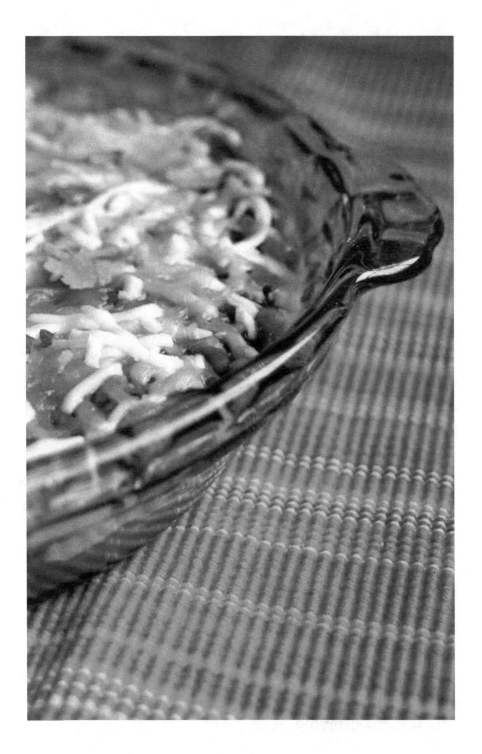

# Air Fryer Beef Casserole

**Serves:** 4

**Cooking Time:** 30 minutes

**Ingredients:**

- 1 green bell pepper, seeded and chopped
- 1 onion, chopped
- 1-pound ground beef /450G
- 3 cloves of garlic, minced
- 3 tablespoons essential olive oil /45ML
- 6 cups eggs, beaten
- Salt and pepper to taste

**Instructions:**

1) Preheat mid-air fryer for 5 minutes.
2) Mix the bottom beef, onion, garlic, organic olive oil, and bell pepper in a baking pan. Season with salt and pepper to taste.
3) Pour inside the beaten eggs and mix properly.
4) Place the pan in a mid-air fryer.
5) Bake for 30 Minutes at 325° F or 163°C .

**Nutrition information:**

- Calories per serving: 1520
- Carbohydrates: 10.4g

- Protein: 87.9g
- Fat: 125.11g

# Almond Flour 'n Egg Crusted Beef

**Serves:** 1

**Cooking Time:** 15

**Ingredients:**

- ½ cup almond flour /65G
- 1 egg, beaten
- 1 slice of lemon, to offer
- 1/2-pound beef schnitzel /225G
- 2 tablespoons vegetable oil /30ML

**Instructions:**

1) Preheat mid-air fryer for 5 minutes.
2) Mix the oil and almond flour.
3) Dip the schnitzel in the egg and then turnover in the almond flour mixture.
4) Turnover the beef in the almond flour mix.
5) Place in the air fryer and cook for 15 minutes at 350° F or 177°C .
6) Serve with a slice of lemon.

**Nutrition information:**

- Calories per serving: 732
- Carbohydrates: 1.1g
- Protein: 55.6g

- Fat: 56.1g

# Another Easy Teriyaki BBQ Recipe

**Servings per Recipe:** 2

**Cooking Time:** 15

## Ingredients:

- 1 tbsp honey /15ML
- 1 tbsp mirin /15ML
- 1 tbsp soy sauce /15ML
- 1 thumb-sized little bit of fresh ginger, grated
- 14 oz lean diced steak, with fat trimmed /420G

## Instructions:

1) Mix all ingredients in a bowl and marinate for about an hour. Turning over halfway through marinating time.
2) Skewer the mead and place it on the skewer rack.
3) Cook for 5 minutes at 390° F or 199°C or desired doneness.
4) Serve and enjoy.

## Nutrition Information:

- Calories per Serving: 460
- Carbs: 10.6g
- Protein: 55.8g
- Fat: 21.6g

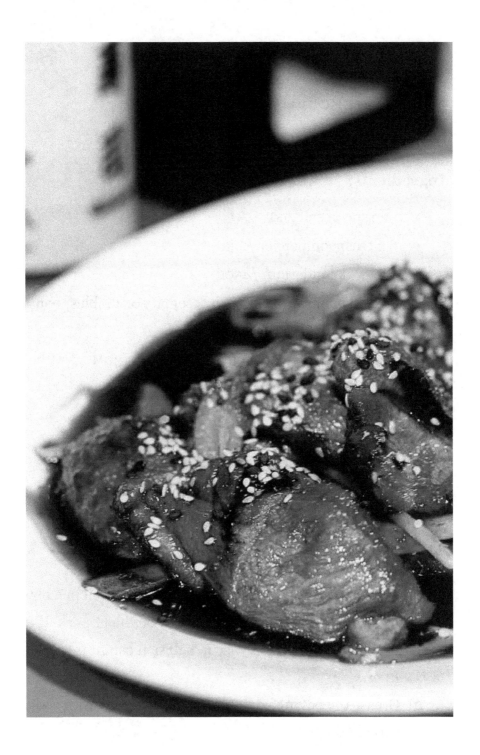

# Apricot Glazed Pork Tenderloins

**Servings per Recipe:** 3

**Cooking Time:** 30 Minutes

**Ingredients:**

- 1 teaspoon salt /5G
- 1/2 teaspoon pepper /2.5G
- 1-lb pork tenderloin /450G
- 2 tablespoons minced fresh rosemary or 1 tablespoon dried rosemary, crushed /30G
- 2 tablespoons organic olive oil, divided /30ML
- 4 garlic cloves, minced

- Apricot Glaze Ingredients

- 1 cup apricot preserves /130G
- 2 garlic cloves, minced
- 3 tablespoons fresh lemon juice /45ML

**Instructions:**

1) Mix pepper, salt, garlic, oil, and rosemary well in a bowl. Brush the mixed seasoning lavishly on the ut pork. If needed cut pork crosswise in half so it can fit into the air fryer.
2) Grease the baking pan of the air fryer lightly with cooking spray. Add pork.

3) Place in the preheated 390° F or 199°C air fryer for 3 minutes and allow the pork to brown on both sides.
4) Mix all glaze ingredients well in a small bowl. Baste pork every 5 minutes.
5) Cook for 20 Minutes at 330° F or 166°C .
6) Serve and enjoy

## Nutrition Information:

- Calories per Serving: 281
- Carbs: 27.0g
- Protein: 23.0g
- Fat: 9.0g

# Baby Back Rib Recipe from Kansas City

**Servings per Recipe:** 2

**Cooking Time:** 50 minutes

**Ingredients:**

- ¼ cup using apple cider vinegar /62.5ML
- ¼ cup molasses /32.5G
- ¼ teaspoon cayenne /1.25G
- 1 cup ketchup /250ML
- 1 tablespoon brown sugar /15G
- 1 tablespoon liquid smoke seasoning, hickory /15ML
- 1 tablespoon Worcestershire sauce /15ML
- 1 teaspoon dry mustard /15G
- 1-pound pork ribs, small /15G
- 2 cloves of garlic
- Salt and pepper to taste

**Instructions:**

1) Place all ingredients in a Ziploc bag and allow to marinate in the fridge for some hours.
2) Preheat mid-air fryer to 390° F or 199°C .
3) Place the grill pan in the air fryer.
4) Grill meat for 25 minutes per batch.
5) Flip the meat halfway through the cooking time.

6) Pour the marinade into a saucepan and allow it to simmer and thicken.

7) Pour the thicken marinade in the meat before serving.

## Nutrition information:

- Calories per serving: 634
- Carbs: 32g
- Protein: 32g
- Fat: 42g

# Easy & The Traditional Beef Roast Recipe

**Serves:** 12

**Cooking Time:** 120 minutes

## Ingredients:

- 1 cup organic beef broth /250ML
- 3 pounds beef round roast /1350G
- 4 tablespoons essential olive oil /60ML
- Salt and pepper to taste

## Instructions:

1) Put all ingredients in a Ziploc bag, allow to marinate in the fridge for 2 hours.
2) Preheat mid-air fryer for 5 minutes.
3) Transfer all ingredients to a baking dish that may fit in the air fryer.
4) Place in the air fryer and cook for 2 hours for 400° F or 205°C .

## Nutrition information:

- Calories per serving: 284
- Carbohydrates:0.4 g
- Protein: 23.7g
- Fat: 20.8g

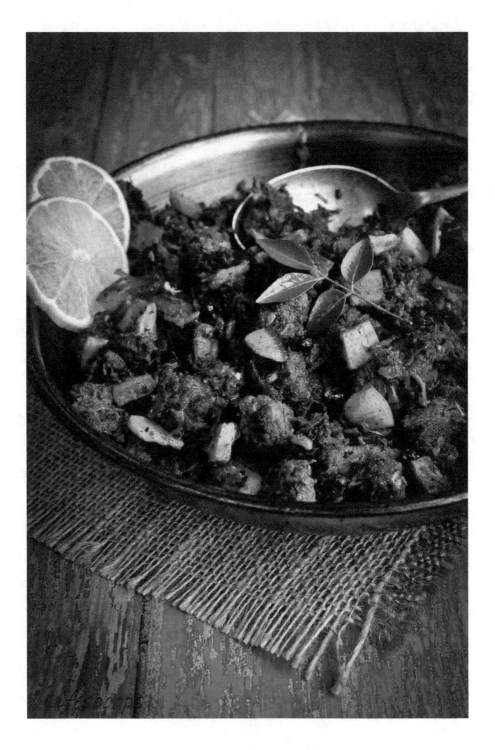

# Easy Corn Dog Bites

**Servings per Recipe:** 2

**Cooking Time:** 10

## Ingredients:

- ½ cup all-purpose flour /65G
- 1 ½ cup crushed cornflakes /195G
- 2 large beef sausages, cut by 50 per cent crosswise
- 2 large eggs, beaten
- Salt and pepper to taste

## Instructions

1) Preheat the air fryer to 330° F or 166°C .
2) Skewer the sausages with a mental skewer that came with the double layer rack accessory.
3) In a mixing bowl, combine the flour and eggs to create a batter. Season with salt and pepper to taste. Add water if too dry.
4) Dip the skewered sausages in the batter and dredge in cornflakes.
5) Place in the double layer rack and cook for 10 minutes.

## Nutrition information:

- Calories per serving: 79

- Carbs:8 g
- Protein: 5g
- Fat: 3g

# Egg Noodles, Ground Beef & Tomato Sauce Bake

**Servings per Recipe:** 3

**Cooking Time:** 45 minutes

## Ingredients:

- 1 (15 ounces) can tomato sauce /450ML
- 4-ounce egg noodles, cooked according to manufacturer's directions /120G
- 1/2-pound ground beef /225G
- 1/2 teaspoon white sugar /2.5G
- 1/2 teaspoon salt /2.5G
- 1/2 teaspoon garlic salt /2.5G
- 1/2 cup sour cream /125ML
- 1/2 large white onion, diced
- 1/4 cup shredded sharp Cheddar cheese, or higher to taste /32.5G
- 1.5-ounce cream cheese /45G

## Instructions:

1) Grease the baking pan of the air fryer lightly with cooking spray. Add ground beef, for 10 minutes cook on 360° F or 183°C . Halfway through cooking time crush beef.
2) When done cooking, remove excess fat.

3) Stir in tomato sauce, garlic salt, salt, and sugar. Mix well and cook for the next 15 minutes. Transfer to a bowl.

4) Whisk onion, cream cheese, and sour cream properly in a bowl.

5) Place half of the egg noodles on the bottom of the air fryer baking pan. Top with 50 % of the sour cream mixture, then half the tomato sauce mixture. Repeat layering. And then top of with cheese.

6) Cover the pan with foil.

7) Cook for the next 15 minutes. Uncover and cook for the next 5 minutes.

8) Serve and enjoy

## Nutrition Information:

- Calories per Serving: 524
- Carbs: 39.4g
- Protein: 24.5g
- Fat: 29.8g

# Eggs 'n Bacon on Biscuit Brekky

**Servings per Recipe:** 4

**Cooking Time:** 28 minutes

**Ingredients:**

- ¼ cup milk /62.5ML
- ½ of 16-ounces refrigerated breakfast biscuits /240G
- 1 cup shredded extra-sharp cheddar cheese /130G
- 4 scallions, chopped
- 5 eggs
- 8 slices cooked center cut bacon

**Instructions:**

1) Set the pan over heat and cook for 8 minutes at 360° F or 183°C or until crisped. Remove bacon and discard excess fat.
2) Evenly spread biscuits on the bottom of the basket. For 5 minutes, cook at 360° F or 183°C .
3) Meanwhile, whisk eggs, milk, and scallions in a bowl.
4) Remove basket, evenly layer bacon ahead of biscuit, sprinkle cheese on top, and pour eggs.
5) Cook for 15 minutes or until eggs are set.
6) Serve and enjoy

**Nutrition Information:**

- Calories per Serving: 241
- Carbs: 4.3g
- Protein: 22.6g
- Fat: 23.7g

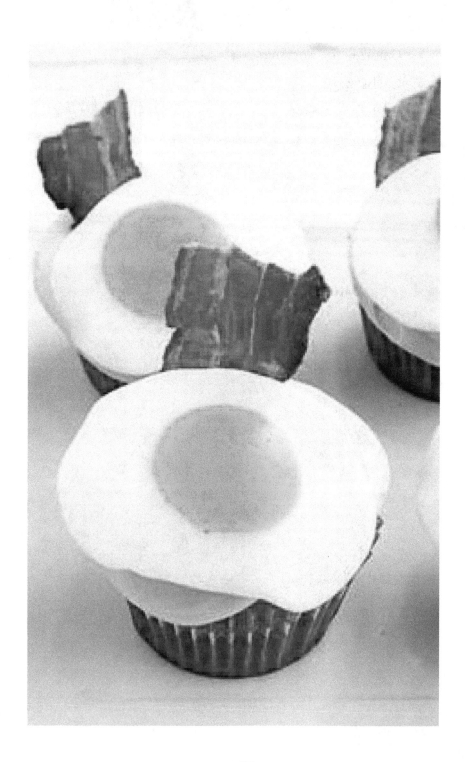

# Fat Burger Bombs

**Serves:** 6

**Cooking Time:** 20 Minutes

**Ingredients:**

- ½ pound ground beef /225G
- 1 cup almond flour /130G
- 12 slices uncured bacon, chopped
- 2 eggs, beaten
- 3 tablespoons olive oil /45ML
- Salt and pepper to taste

**Instructions:**

1) In a mixing bowl, combine all ingredients aside from the olive oil.
2) Use your hands to make small balls with the mixture. Place in the baking sheet and allow to marinate and put in the fridge for about 2 hours.
3) Preheat mid-air fryer for 5 minutes.
4) Brush the meatballs with olive oil on all sides.
5) Place in the air fryer basket.
6) Cook for 20 minutes at 350° F or 177°C .
7) Halfway through the cooking time, shake the fryer basket for a more even cooking.

**Nutrition information:**

- Calories per serving: 412
- Carbohydrates: 1.5g
- Protein: 19.2g
- Fat: 36.6g

# Rib Eye Steak Recipe from Hawaii

**Servings per Recipe:** 6

**Cooking Time:** 45 minutes

**Ingredients:**

- ½ cup soy sauce /125ML
- ½ cup sugar /65G
- 1-inch ginger, grated
- 2 cups pineapple juice /500ML
- 2 teaspoons sesame oil /10ML
- 3 pounds rib-eye steaks /1350G
- 5 tablespoons using apple cider vinegar /75ML

**Instructions:**

1) Add all ingredients in a Ziploc bag and allow to marinate in the fridge for about 120 minutes.
2) Preheat mid-air fryer to 390° F or 199°C .
3) Place the grill pan accessory in the air fryer.
4) Grill the meat for 15 minutes. Flip every 8 minutes and cook in batches if needed.
5) Meanwhile, pour the marinade inside a saucepan and allow simmer before the sauce thickens.
6) Brush the grilled meat using the sauce before serving.

**Nutrition information:**

- Calories per serving: 612
- Carbs: 28g
- Protein: 44g
- Fat: 36g

# Rib Eye Steak Seasoned with Italian Herb

**Servings per Recipe:** 4

**Cooking Time:** 45 minutes

## Ingredients

- 1 packet Italian herb mix
- 1 tablespoon olive oil /15ML
- 2 pounds bone-in rib-eye steak /900G
- Salt and pepper to taste

## Instructions:

1) Preheat air fryer to 390° F or 199°C .
2) Place the grill pan accessory in the mid-air fryer.
3) Season the steak with salt, pepper, Italian herb mix, and extra virgin olive oil. Cover top with foil.
4) Grill for 45 minutes and flip the steak halfway over the cooking time.

## Nutrition information:

- Calories per serving: 481
- Carbs:1.1 g
- Protein: 50.9g
- Fat: 30.3g

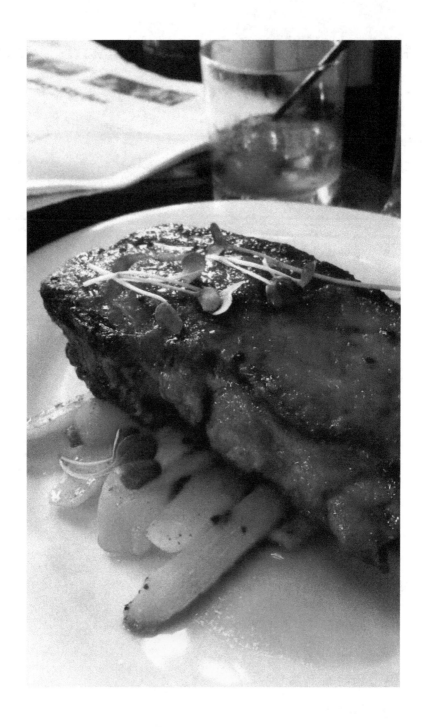

# Roast Beef with Balsamic-Honey Sauce

**Serves:** 10

**Cooking Time:** a couple of hours

**Ingredients:**

- ½ cup balsamic vinegar /65ML
- ½ teaspoon red pepper flakes /2.5G
- 1 cup beef organic beef broth /250ML
- 1 tablespoon coconut aminos /15G
- 1 tablespoon honey /15ML
- 1 tablespoon Worcestershire sauce /15ML
- 3 pounds boneless roast beef /1350G
- 4 cloves of garlic, minced
- 4 tablespoons essential olive oil /60ML

**Instructions:**

1) Fill up the entire bottom of the baking dish with all ingredients.
2) Place in the air fryer. Close.
3) Cook for 120 minutes at 400° F or 205°C .

**Nutrition information:**

- Calories per serving: 325
- Carbohydrates: 6.9g
- Protein: 36.2g

- Fat: 16.9g

# Roast Beef with Buttered Garlic-Celery

**Serves:** 8

**Cooking Time:** 60 minutes

**Ingredients:**

- 1 bulb of garlic, peeled and crushed
- 1 tablespoon butter  /15G
- 2 medium onions, chopped
- 2 pounds topside of beef /900G
- 2 sticks of celery, sliced
- 3 tablespoons essential olive oil /45ML
- A couple of fresh herbs of your choice
- Salt and pepper to taste

**Instructions:**

1) Preheat mid-air fryer for 5 minutes.
2) Put all of the ingredients in a baking dish and stir properly.
3) Place the dish in a mid-air fryer and bake for one hour at 350° F or 177°C .

**Nutrition information:**

- Calories per serving: 243
- Carbohydrates: 3.1g
- Protein: 16.7g

- Fat: 18.2g

# Roasted Ribeye Steak with Rum

**Servings per Recipe:** 4

**Cooking Time:** 50 minutes

**Ingredients:**

- ½ cup rum /125ML
- 2 pounds bone-in ribeye steak /900G
- 2 tablespoons extra virgin olive oil /30ML
- Salt and black pepper to taste

**Instructions:**

1) Place all ingredients in a Ziploc bag and allow to marinate in the fridge for about an hour.
2) Preheat mid-air fryer to 390° F or 199°C .
3) Place the grill pan accessory in the air fryer.
4) Grill for 25 minutes per piece.
5) Flip the meat every 10 minutes.

**Nutrition information:**

- Calories per serving: 390
- Carbs: 0.1g
- Protein: 48.9g
- Fat: 21.5g

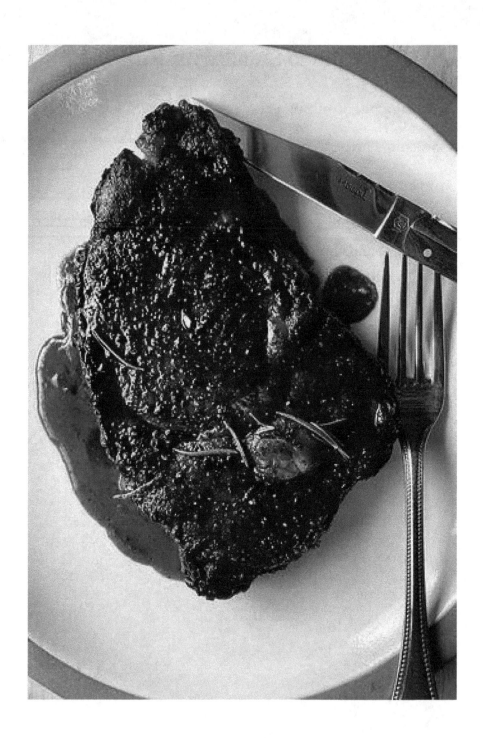

# Easy Chicken Fried Rice

**Servings per Recipe:** 3

**Cooking Time:** 20 Minutes

**Ingredients:**

- 1 cup frozen peas & carrots /130G
- 1 packed cup cooked chicken, diced
- 1 tbsp vegetable oil /15ML
- 1/2 cup onion, diced /65G
- 3 cups cold cooked white rice /390G
- 6 tbsp soy sauce /90ML

**Instructions:**

1) With vegetable oil lightly grease the baking pan of the air fryer. Add frozen carrots and peas.
2) Cook at 360° F or 183°C for 5 minutes.
3) Stir in the chicken and cook for an additional 5 minutes.
4) Add the remaining ingredients and mix well to combine.
5) Cook for an additional 10 minutes. Mix after 5 minutes.
6) Serve and enjoy.

**Nutrition Information:**

- Calories per Serving: 445
- Carbs: 59.4g
- Protein: 20.0g

- Fat: 14.1g

# Easy Fried Chicken Southern Style

**Serves:** 6

**Cooking Time:** 30 Minutes

**Ingredients:**

- 1 cup coconut flour /130G
- 1 teaspoon garlic powder /5G
- 1 teaspoon paprika  /5G
- 1 teaspoon pepper /5G
- 1 teaspoon salt /5G
- 5 pounds chicken leg quarters /2250G

**Instructions:**

1) Preheat mid-air fryer for 5 minutes.
2) Add all ingredients to a bowl and give a stir.
3) Place ingredients in the air fryer.
4) Cook for 30 minutes at 350° F or 177°C .

**Nutrition information:**

- Calories per serving:611
- Carbohydrates: 2.8g
- Protein: 92.7g
- Fat: 25.4g

# Easy How-To Hard Boil Egg in Air Fryer

**Serves:** 6

**Cooking Time:** 15

**Ingredients:**

- 6 eggs

**Instructions:**

1) Preheat the air fryer for 5 minutes.
2) Place the eggs in the air fryer basket.
3) Cook for 15 minutes at 360° F or 183°C .
4) Remove from air fryer basket and place in cold water.

**Nutrition information:**

- Calories per serving: 140
- Carbohydrates: 0g
- Protein: 12g
- Fat: 10g

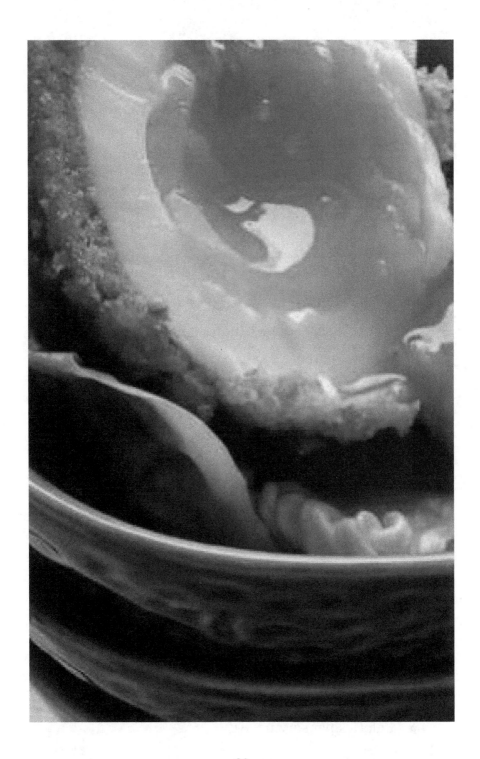

# Eggs 'n Turkey Bake

**Serves:** 4

**Cooking Time:** 15 minutes

**Ingredients:**

- ½ teaspoon garlic powder /2.5G
- ½ teaspoon onion powder /2.5G
- 1 cup coconut milk /250ML
- 1-pound leftover turkey, shredded /450G
- 2 cups kale, chopped /260G
- 4 eggs, beaten
- Salt and pepper to taste

**Instructions:**

1) Preheat the air fryer for 5 minutes.
2) Add the eggs, coconut milk, garlic powder, and onion powder to a bowl and mix. Season with salt and pepper to taste.
3) Place the turkey meat and kale in the baking dish.
4) Pour in the egg mixture.
5) Place inside the air fryer.
6) Cook for 15 minutes at 350° F or 177°C .

**Nutrition information:**

- Calories per serving: 817

- Carbohydrates: 3.6g
- Protein: 32.9g
- Fat: 74.5g

# Eggs Benedict on English Muffins

**Servings per Recipe:** 5

**Cooking Time:** 40 minutes

## Ingredients:

- ½ tsp onion powder /2.5G
- 1 cup milk /250ML
- 1 stalk green onions, chopped
- 1/2 (.9 ounce) package hollandaise sauce mix
- 1/2 cup milk /125ML
- 1/2 teaspoon salt / 2.5G
- 1/4 teaspoon paprika /1.25G
- 2 tablespoons margarine /30G
- 3 English muffins, cut into 1/2-inch dice
- 4 large eggs
- 6-ounces Canadian bacon, cut into 1/2-inch dice /180G

## Instructions:

1) Lightly oil the baking pan of the air fryer with cooking spray.
2) Arrange half of the bacon at bottom of the pan, Spread the dried English muffins on top. Also, spread the remaining bacon at the top.

3) Whisk the eggs, 1 cup milk, green onions, onion powder and salt well in a bowl. Pour over the English muffin mixture. Sprinkle paprika on top. Cover with foil and refrigerate overnight.

4) Preheat air fryer to 390° F or 199°C .

5) Cook in the air fryer for 25 minutes. Remove foil and continue cooking for another 15 minutes or until set.

6) Meanwhile, make the hollandaise sauce by melting margarine in a sauce pan. Mix remaining milk and hollandaise sauce in a small bowl and whisk into melted margarine. Stir continuously and simmer until thickened.

7) Serve with sauce and enjoy.

## Nutrition Information:

- Calories per Serving: 282
- Carbs: 21.2g
- Protein: 17.5g
- Fat: 14.1g

# Melts in Your Mouth Caramel Cheesecake

**Servings per Recipe:** 8

**Cooking Time:** 40 minutes

**Ingredients:**

- 1 Can Dulce de Leche
- 1 Tbsp Melted Chocolate /15ML
- 1 Tbsp Vanilla Essence /15ML
- 250 g Caster Sugar
- 4 Large Eggs
- 50 g Melted Butter
- 500 g Soft Cheese
- 6 Digestives, crumbled

**Instructions:**

1) Grease baking pan of air fryer with oil using cooking spray. Mix and press to crush. Add melted butter to the pan. Spread dulce de leche.
2) Beat soft cheese and sugar until fluffy. Stir in vanilla and egg. Pour mixture over dulce de leche.
3) Cover pan with foil. Cook for 15 minutes at 390° F or 199°C .

4) Reduce to 330° F or 166°C and cook for 10 minutes. Reduce to 300° F or 149°C and cook for 15 minutes.

5) Open the air fryer and allow to cool. After which, place in the refrigerator for 4 hours before slicing.

6) Serve and enjoy.

## Nutrition Information:

- Calories per Serving: 463
- Carbs: 44.1g
- Protein: 17.9g
- Fat: 23.8g

# Mouth-Watering Strawberry Cobbler

**Servings per Recipe:** 4

**Cooking Time:** 25 minutes

**Ingredients:**

- tablespoon butter, diced /15G
- tablespoon and two teaspoons butter /25G
- 1-1/2 teaspoons cornstarch /7.5G
- 1/2 cup water /125ML
- 1-1/2 cups strawberries, hulled /195G
- 1/2 cup all-purpose flour /65G
- 1-1/2 teaspoons white sugar /7.5G
- 1/4 cup white sugar /32.5G
- 1/4 teaspoon salt /1.25G
- 1/4 cup heavy whipping cream /62.5ML
- 3/4 teaspoon baking powder /3.75G

**Instructions:**

1) Grease baking pan of air fryer with oil using cooking spray. Add water, cornstarch, and sugar. Cook for 10 minutes at 390° F or 199°C or until hot and thick. Add strawberries and mix well. Dress tops with 1 tbsp butter.

2) Mix salt, baking powder, sugar, and flour. Cut in 1 tbsp and two tsp butter. Mix in cream. Mix in the berries.

3) Cook for 15 minutes at 390° F or 199°C , until tops are lightly browned.

4) Serve and enjoy.

## Nutrition Information:

- Calories per Serving: 255
- Carbs: 32.0g
- Protein: 2.4g
- Fat: 13.0g

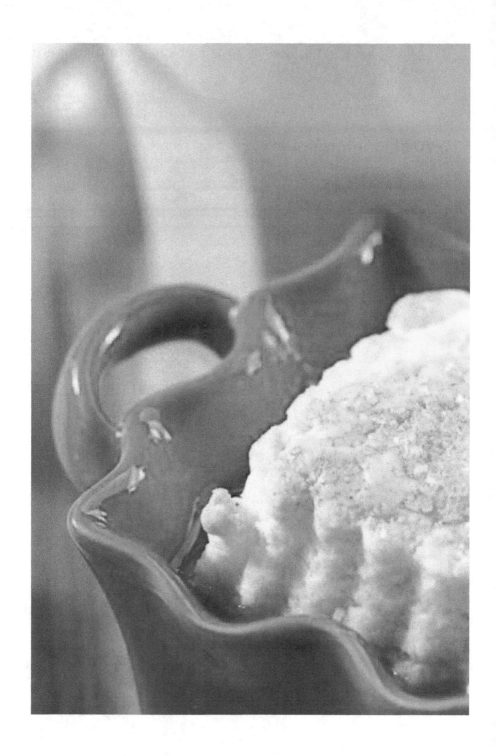

# Oriental Coconut Cake

**Servings per Recipe:** 8

**Cooking Time:** 40 minutes

**Ingredients:**

- 1 cup gluten-free flour /130G
- 2 eggs
- 1/2 cup flaked coconut /65G
- 1-1/2 teaspoons baking powder /7.5G
- 1/2 teaspoon baking soda /2.5G
- 1/2 teaspoon xanthan gum /2.5G
- 1/2 teaspoon salt /2.5G
- 1/2 cup coconut milk /125ML
- 1/2 cup vegetable oil /125ML
- 1/2 teaspoon vanilla flavor /2.5ML
- 1/4 cup chopped walnuts /32.5G
- 3/4 cup white sugar /98G

**Instructions:**

1) Blend all wet ingredients. Add dry ingredients and blend thoroughly.
2) Grease baking pan of air fryer lightly with oil using cooking spray.
3) Pour in batter. Cover pan with foil.
4) Cook for 30 minutes at 330° F or 166°C .

5) Let it rest for 10 Minutes

6) Serve and enjoy.

## Nutrition Information:

- Calories per Serving: 359
- Carbs: 35.2g
- Protein: 4.3g
- Fat: 22.3g

# Pecan-Cranberry Cake

**Servings per Recipe:** 6

**Cooking Time:** 25 minutes

**Ingredients:**

- 1 1/2 cups Almond Flour /195G
- 1 tsp baking powder /5G
- 1/2 cup fresh cranberries /65G
- 1/2 tsp vanilla extract /2.5ML
- 1/4 cup cashew milk (or use any dairy or non-dairy milk you like) /62.5ML
- 1/4 cup chopped pecans /32.5G
- 1/4 cup Monk fruit (or make use of preferred sweetener) /32.5G
- 1/4 tsp cinnamon /1.25G
- 1/8 tsp salt /0.625G
- 2 large eggs

**Instructions:**

1) Blend all wet ingredients and mix well. Add all dry ingredients except for cranberries and pecans. Blend well until smooth.
2) Grease baking pan of air fryer with cooking spray. Pour in batter. Sprinkle cranberries and pecans at the top.
3) For twenty minutes, cook on 330° F or 166°C .

4) Allow to sit for 5 minutes.

5) Serve and enjoy

## Nutrition Information:

- Calories per Serving: 98
- Carbs: 11.7g
- Protein: 1.7g
- Fat: 4.9g

# Poppy Seed Pound Cake

**Serves:** 8

**Cooking Time:** 20 Minutes

## Ingredients

- ¼ cup erythritol powder /32.5G
- ¼ teaspoon vanilla flavor /1.25ML
- ½ cup coconut milk /125ML
- 1 ½ cups almond flour /195G
- 1 ½ teaspoon baking powder /7.5G
- 1/3 cup butter, unsalted /83G
- 2 large eggs, beaten
- 2 tablespoon psyllium husk powder /30G
- 2 tablespoons poppy seeds /30G

## Instructions:

1) Preheat the air fryer for 5 minutes.
2) Combine all ingredients and mix well.
3) Use a hand mixer to mix everything.
4) Pour into a small loaf pan that may easily fit in a mid-air fryer.
5) Bake for 20 minutes at 375° F or 191°C or if a toothpick comes clean after inserted in the middle.

## Nutrition information:

- Calories per serving: 145
- Carbohydrates: 3.6
- Protein: 2.1g
- Fat: 13.6g

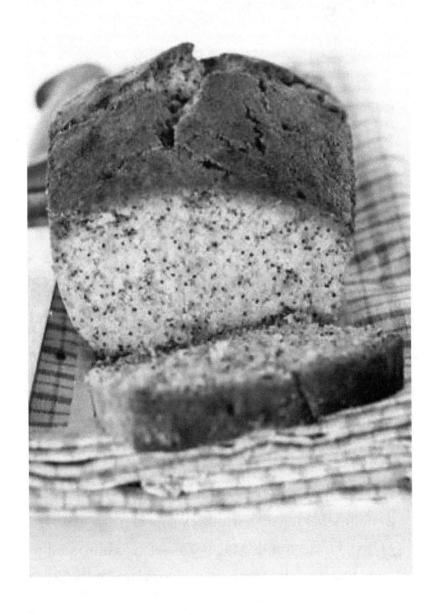

# Zucchini-Choco Bread

**Serves:** 12

**Cooking Time:** 20 minutes

**Ingredients:**

- ¼ teaspoon salt /1.25G
- ½ cup almond milk /125ML
- ½ cup maple syrup /125ML
- ½ cup sunflower oil /125ML
- ½ cup unsweetened powdered cocoa /65G
- 1 cup oat flour /130G
- 1 cup zucchini, shredded and squeezed /250ML
- ·1 tablespoon flax egg (1 tablespoon or 15ML flax meal + 3 tablespoons or 45ML water)
- 1 teaspoon using apple cider vinegar /5ML
- 1 teaspoon baking soda /5G
- 1 teaspoon vanilla extract /5G
- 1/3 cup chocolate chips /43G

**Instructions:**

1) Preheat the air fryer to 350° F or 177°C .
2) Line a baking dish with wax paper.
3) In a bowl, combine the flax meal, zucchini, sunflower oil, maple, vanilla, apple cider vinegar and milk. Mix well.

4) Add oat flour, baking soda, hot chocolate mix, and salt. Mix until well combined.
5) Add the chocolate chips.
6) Pour the mixture inside a baking dish and cook for 15 minutes or until a toothpick inserted in the middle comes out clean.

## Nutrition information:

- Calories per serving: 213
- Carbohydrates:24.2 g
- Protein: 4.6g
- Fat: 10.9g